AUTOIMMUNE HEPATITIS DISEASE

Understanding, Treating, and Managing a Chronic Liver Condition

DR. MATAMI JAMES

Copyright ©2023by Dr. Matami James

All rights reserved. No part of this publication may be reproduced, distributed, or transmitted in any form or by any means, including photocopying, recording, or other electronic or mechanical methods, without the prior written permission of the publisher, except in the case of brief quotations embodied in critical reviews and certain other noncommercial uses permitted by copyright law

CONTENTS

CHAPTER 1

Introduction to Autoimmune Hepatitis Disease

Autoimmune hepatitis disease is a chronic and progressive liver disorder that affects millions of people worldwide. In this chapter, we will explore the definition, historical background, and scope of this disease.

1.1 Definition and Explanation of Autoimmune Hepatitis Disease

Autoimmune hepatitis disease is a condition in which the body's immune system attacks the liver cells, leading to inflammation and damage. The disease can occur at any age but is more common in women than men. There are two types of autoimmune hepatitis disease - type 1 and type 2 - which are classified based on the presence of certain autoantibodies in the blood.

The exact cause of autoimmune hepatitis disease is unknown, but genetic and environmental factors are believed to play a role.

Common risk factors include a family history of the disease, exposure to certain drugs or toxins, viral infections, and autoimmune disorders.

Symptoms of autoimmune hepatitis disease can be mild or severe and may include fatigue, abdominal discomfort, jaundice, and loss of appetite. The disease can also lead to complications such as cirrhosis, liver failure, and liver cancer.

1.2 Historical Background and Discovery

The first case of autoimmune hepatitis disease was reported in 1950 by a physician named Waldenström, who described a group of patients with chronic liver inflammation and autoantibodies in their blood. Over the years, researchers have made significant progress in understanding the disease's pathophysiology, diagnosis, and treatment.

In the 1960s, researchers identified a specific type of autoantibody called antinuclear antibody (ANA) that is present in many patients with autoimmune hepatitis disease. In the 1970s, a diagnostic scoring system was developed that allowed doctors to assess the severity of the disease and monitor patients' response to treatment.

In recent years, advances in genetic testing and immunology have led to a better understanding of the underlying mechanisms of autoimmune hepatitis disease. However, there is still much to learn about the disease's complex pathophysiology and optimal treatment strategies.

1.3 Scope and Significance of the Disease

Autoimmune hepatitis disease is a significant public health problem, with an estimated 2-3 million people affected worldwide. The disease can cause significant morbidity and mortality, and early diagnosis and treatment are critical for improving patients' outcomes.

Despite the availability of effective treatments, many patients with autoimmune hepatitis disease continue to experience chronic liver inflammation and progression to cirrhosis, liver failure, and liver cancer.

There is a need for further research to improve our understanding of the disease's pathophysiology, identify new therapeutic targets, and develop more effective treatment strategies.

CHAPTER 2

Causes and Risk Factors of Autoimmune Hepatitis Disease

Autoimmune hepatitis disease is a complex condition with multiple underlying causes and risk factors. In this chapter, we will explore the various factors that contribute to the development and progression of this disease.

2.1 Genetics and Family History

Genetics plays a significant role in autoimmune hepatitis disease, and there is a strong link between the disease and certain human leukocyte antigen (HLA) genes. Studies have shown that individuals with specific HLA alleles, such as HLA-DR3, HLA-DR4, and HLA-DRB1, are at an increased risk of developing autoimmune hepatitis disease.

Family history is another important risk factor, as the disease is more common among individuals with relatives who have been diagnosed with autoimmune diseases or liver disorders.

2.2 Environmental Factors

Environmental factors, such as exposure to certain drugs and toxins, can trigger autoimmune hepatitis disease in genetically susceptible individuals. Medications such as nitrofurantoin, minocycline, and methyldopa have been implicated in the development of autoimmune hepatitis disease.

Other environmental factors that may contribute to the disease include exposure to viruses, bacteria, and other infectious agents. In particular, hepatitis C virus (HCV) infection has been linked to the development of autoimmune hepatitis disease.

2.3 Infections and Triggers

Infections can trigger autoimmune hepatitis disease in susceptible individuals, especially in those who have a genetic predisposition to the disease. Viral infections such as hepatitis A, B, and C, as well as cytomegalovirus (CMV) and Epstein-Barr virus (EBV), have been linked to the development of autoimmune hepatitis disease.

Other triggers that can exacerbate the disease include alcohol, obesity, and certain autoimmune disorders such as rheumatoid arthritis, lupus, and thyroiditis.

2.4 Other Risk Factors and Contributing Factors

Other risk factors that may contribute to the development of autoimmune hepatitis disease include gender, age, and race. Women are more likely to develop the disease than men, and the disease is most commonly diagnosed in individuals between the ages of 15 and 40. Certain ethnic groups, such as Hispanics and Caucasians, are also at an increased risk of developing the disease.

Other contributing factors that may play a role in the development of autoimmune hepatitis disease include imbalances in the gut microbiome, stress, and hormonal changes.

In conclusion, autoimmune hepatitis disease is a multifactorial condition with multiple underlying causes and risk factors. A better understanding of these factors is crucial for the development of effective prevention and treatment strategies.

CHAPTER 3

Symptoms and Diagnosis of Autoimmune Hepatitis Disease

Autoimmune hepatitis disease is a chronic liver disorder that can be difficult to diagnose due to its varied and nonspecific symptoms. In this chapter, we will explore the different types of autoimmune hepatitis disease, the common symptoms and signs, and the diagnostic procedures used to confirm a diagnosis.

3.1 Types of Autoimmune Hepatitis Disease

There are two main types of autoimmune hepatitis disease: type 1 and type 2. Type 1 is the most common form of the disease and is characterized by the presence of antibodies against smooth muscle (SMA) and/or liver/kidney microsomes (LKM). Type 2 is less common and is characterized by the presence of antibodies against liver/kidney microsomes type 1 (LKM-1) and/or liver cytosol type 1 (LC-1).

3.2 Symptoms and Signs

The symptoms of autoimmune hepatitis disease can vary widely, and some patients may be asymptomatic for a long period of time. Common symptoms and signs include:

- Fatigue

- Abdominal discomfort or pain

- Jaundice

- Itching

- Nausea and vomiting

- Loss of appetite

- Joint pain or swelling

- Spider angiomas (small, red, spider-like blood vessels on the skin)

In some cases, autoimmune hepatitis disease may present with acute symptoms, such as fever, abdominal pain, and an enlarged liver. This is known as acute autoimmune hepatitis and can rapidly progress to liver failure if left untreated.

3.3 Laboratory Tests and Imaging Studies

Laboratory tests and imaging studies are essential for the diagnosis of autoimmune hepatitis disease. Blood tests can detect the presence of autoantibodies, elevated liver enzymes, and signs of liver inflammation. Imaging studies, such as ultrasound, CT scan, or MRI, can also help to identify liver damage and rule out other liver diseases.

3.4 Diagnostic Criteria and Procedures

The diagnosis of autoimmune hepatitis disease is based on a combination of clinical findings, laboratory results, and imaging studies. The diagnostic criteria for autoimmune hepatitis disease include the presence of autoantibodies, elevated liver enzymes, and evidence of liver inflammation on liver biopsy.

Liver biopsy is the gold standard for diagnosing autoimmune hepatitis disease, as it can provide a detailed assessment of the degree of liver damage and the presence of inflammation and fibrosis.

In conclusion, the diagnosis of autoimmune hepatitis disease can be challenging due to its varied and nonspecific symptoms. A thorough evaluation, including laboratory tests, imaging studies, and liver biopsy, is necessary for an accurate diagnosis. Early detection and treatment are crucial for preventing the progression of the disease and minimizing the risk of complications.

CHAPTER 4

Treatment and Management of Autoimmune Hepatitis Disease

Autoimmune hepatitis disease is a chronic autoimmune disorder that requires long-term management to prevent complications and maintain liver function. In this chapter, we will discuss the various treatment options available for autoimmune hepatitis disease, including medications, lifestyle modifications, surgery, and alternative therapies.

4.1 Medications and Drugs Used for Treatment

The mainstay of treatment for autoimmune hepatitis disease is medication to suppress the immune system and reduce liver inflammation. The most commonly used medications for autoimmune hepatitis disease include:

- Corticosteroids: These drugs, such as prednisone and budesonide, are used to reduce inflammation and suppress the immune system.

- Azathioprine: This immunosuppressant drug is often used in combination with corticosteroids to maintain remission and reduce the risk of relapse.

- Mycophenolate mofetil: This medication is an alternative to azathioprine and is used for patients who cannot tolerate or do not respond to azathioprine.

The goal of medication therapy is to induce remission and maintain it over the long term. Patients must be monitored closely for side effects and may require adjustments to their medication regimen over time.

4.2 Diet and Lifestyle Modifications

In addition to medication therapy, diet and lifestyle modifications can help manage autoimmune hepatitis disease. Patients are advised to avoid alcohol and to maintain a healthy weight through a balanced diet and regular exercise. In some cases, a low-salt diet may be recommended to reduce fluid retention and swelling.

Patients should also take steps to reduce stress and get adequate rest, as stress and fatigue can worsen autoimmune symptoms.

4.3 Surgery and Liver Transplantation

In severe cases of autoimmune hepatitis disease, surgery and liver transplantation may be necessary. Surgery may be performed to remove part of the liver or to relieve pressure on the liver caused by an enlarged spleen. Liver transplantation is a treatment option for patients with end-stage liver disease or those who do not respond to medical therapy.

4.4 Alternative and Complementary Therapies

Alternative and complementary therapies, such as herbal supplements, acupuncture, and yoga, may also be used to manage symptoms and improve quality of life. However, it is important to discuss these therapies with a healthcare provider and to use them in conjunction with conventional medical treatment.

In conclusion, autoimmune hepatitis disease is a chronic autoimmune disorder that requires long-term management. Medication therapy, diet and lifestyle modifications, and surgery or liver transplantation may be used to manage symptoms and prevent complications. Patients should work closely with their healthcare providers to develop a personalized

treatment plan and to monitor their condition over
time.

CHAPTER 5

Coping with Autoimmune Hepatitis Disease

Autoimmune hepatitis disease can have a significant impact on a patient's emotional and psychological well-being. In this chapter, we will discuss the emotional and psychological impact of the disease, available support groups and resources, and coping strategies and tips to help patients manage the challenges of living with autoimmune hepatitis disease.

5.1 Emotional and Psychological Impact of the Disease

The diagnosis of a chronic illness such as autoimmune hepatitis disease can be overwhelming and can have a significant impact on a patient's emotional and psychological well-being. Patients may experience a range of emotions, including anger, fear, anxiety, and depression. They may also feel isolated or overwhelmed by the demands of managing their condition.

It is important for patients to recognize the emotional and psychological impact of the disease and to seek support and resources to help them cope.

5.2 Support Groups and Resources

There are many support groups and resources available to help patients with autoimmune hepatitis disease manage the emotional and psychological impact of the disease. These may include:

Support groups: Support groups can provide patients with a safe and supportive environment to share their experiences, connect with others who have similar conditions, and learn coping strategies and tips.

Counseling and therapy: Counseling and therapy can help patients manage the emotional and psychological impact of the disease, learn coping strategies, and improve their overall quality of life.

Online resources: There are many online resources available for patients with autoimmune hepatitis disease, including educational materials, forums, and online support groups.

5.3 Coping Strategies and Tips

In addition to seeking support and resources, there are many coping strategies and tips that can help patients manage the challenges of living with autoimmune hepatitis disease. These may include:

- Learning about the disease: Patients can empower themselves by learning as much as they can about the disease, its symptoms, and treatment options.

- Developing a support system: Patients can reach out to family, friends, and healthcare providers for support and help.

- Staying positive: Staying positive and focusing on the things that bring joy and happiness can help patients manage the emotional and psychological impact of the disease.

- Managing stress: Patients can manage stress through activities such as meditation, deep breathing, or yoga.

- Maintaining a healthy lifestyle: Patients can maintain a healthy lifestyle by following a balanced diet, getting regular exercise, and avoiding alcohol and tobacco.

In conclusion, living with autoimmune hepatitis disease can be challenging, but there are many resources and coping strategies available to help patients manage the emotional and psychological impact of the disease. By seeking support, developing coping strategies, and maintaining a healthy lifestyle, patients can improve their quality of life and manage the challenges of living with autoimmune hepatitis disease.

CHAPTER 6

Prevention and Prognosis

Autoimmune hepatitis disease is a chronic condition that requires ongoing management and monitoring. In this chapter, we will discuss prevention strategies and lifestyle changes, the prognosis and long-term outlook for patients with autoimmune hepatitis disease, and potential complications and risks.

6.1 Prevention Strategies and Lifestyle Changes

There is no known way to prevent autoimmune hepatitis disease, but there are some strategies and lifestyle changes that patients can adopt to help manage the disease and reduce the risk of complications. These may include:

- Maintaining a healthy lifestyle: Patients should aim to maintain a healthy lifestyle by following a balanced diet, getting regular exercise, avoiding alcohol and tobacco, and getting enough rest and sleep.

- Avoiding triggers: Patients should work with their healthcare provider to identify and avoid triggers that can exacerbate their symptoms or cause flare-ups.

- Getting vaccinated: Patients should make sure they are up-to-date on all recommended vaccines, including vaccines for hepatitis A and B.

- Managing other health conditions: Patients with autoimmune hepatitis disease may also have other health conditions that require management, such as diabetes or high blood pressure. It is important for patients to work with their healthcare provider to manage these conditions effectively.

The prognosis for patients with autoimmune hepatitis disease varies depending on the severity of the disease and how quickly it is diagnosed and treated. With proper treatment and management, many patients can achieve remission and lead relatively normal lives.

However, some patients may experience complications or require ongoing treatment to manage their symptoms. In rare cases, the disease can progress to cirrhosis or liver failure, which can be life-threatening.

It is important for patients to work closely with their healthcare provider to monitor their condition and adjust their treatment plan as needed. Regular check-ups and monitoring can help identify any complications early and prevent further damage to the liver.

6.3 Complications and Potential Risks

Complications of autoimmune hepatitis disease may include:

- Cirrhosis: Over time, the inflammation caused by the disease can lead to scarring of the liver, which can progress to cirrhosis.

- Liver failure: In severe cases, autoimmune hepatitis disease can lead to liver failure, which can be life-threatening and may require a liver transplant.

- Increased risk of liver cancer: Patients with cirrhosis or long-standing autoimmune hepatitis disease may be at increased risk of developing liver cancer.

Patients should work closely with their healthcare provider to monitor their condition and manage any complications or potential risks. With proper treatment and management, many patients can achieve remission and lead healthy, productive lives.

CHAPTER 7

Conclusion and Future Directions

In this final chapter, we will summarize the key points discussed in this book, including the causes, symptoms, diagnosis, treatment, and management of autoimmune hepatitis disease. We will also discuss emerging research and future directions for the treatment and management of this condition, and provide some final thoughts and recommendations for patients and healthcare providers.

7.1 Summary of the Book's Content and Key Takeaways

Autoimmune hepatitis disease is a chronic condition that can lead to liver damage and other complications if left untreated. It is caused by an abnormal immune response that targets the liver cells, leading to inflammation and damage.

The symptoms of autoimmune hepatitis disease can vary widely, but may include fatigue, abdominal pain, jaundice, and other symptoms. Diagnosis usually involves a combination of blood tests, imaging studies, and liver biopsy.

Treatment typically involves medications to suppress the immune system and reduce inflammation, as well as lifestyle modifications to support liver health. In severe cases, liver transplantation may be necessary.

The prognosis for patients with autoimmune hepatitis disease varies, but with proper treatment and management, many patients can achieve remission and lead healthy, productive lives.

7.2 Emerging Research and Future Directions for Treatment and Management

While current treatments for autoimmune hepatitis disease are effective for many patients, there is ongoing research aimed at developing new therapies and improving existing ones. Some areas of emerging research include:

- Biomarkers for diagnosis and monitoring: Researchers are exploring new biomarkers that can help diagnose and monitor autoimmune hepatitis disease more accurately and non-invasively.

- New medications and treatment approaches: Researchers are exploring new medications and treatment approaches that can improve outcomes for patients with autoimmune hepatitis disease and reduce the risk of complications.

- Precision medicine: Researchers are exploring the use of precision medicine approaches to tailor treatment plans to individual patients based on their genetic and other characteristics.

7.3 Final Thoughts and Recommendations

Autoimmune hepatitis disease is a serious condition that requires ongoing management and monitoring. Patients should work closely with their healthcare provider to develop a personalized treatment plan that meets their individual needs and goals.

Lifestyle modifications, such as maintaining a healthy diet and getting regular exercise, can also help support liver health and improve overall well-being.

Finally, it is important for patients to stay up-to-date on the latest research and treatment options for autoimmune hepatitis disease, and to work with their healthcare provider to adjust their treatment plan as needed. With ongoing care and management, many patients can achieve remission and lead healthy, productive lives.

www.ingramcontent.com/pod-product-compliance
Lightning Source LLC
Chambersburg PA
CBHW070945250726
48663CB00001B/82